How to Get Pregnant Fast

Understanding Ovulation, Fertility, & Conception – And What You Can Do to Speed Things Up

~ Tips for Getting Pregnant Fast ~

by Makayla Bryson

1

Table of Contents

Introduction

No other phase of life harbors quite as much meaning, effort, reward and a promise of better things – in essence, the hallmarks of positive change – as when you and your partner are ready to step into parenthood.

Now that you've made this decision, and have come to the conclusion that the two of you are mentally, emotionally, and financially ready to expand your own family, you've embarked upon a journey to understand and learn all you can about conception in your keen enthusiasm to have a child – whether you're just eager, or you want the baby to be born at a specific time.

However, while there are plenty of sources of information on the matter – maybe too many – they're often disjointed, abrupt, and hardly possess all the information you need, all in one location. Many such sources leave you more confused than when you started reading; or seem sketchy and circumspect, and leave you wondering as to their validity and authenticity; or perhaps they are just incomplete, thus giving you half-baked information.

But, how do you separate fact from fiction? How can you truly understand the biological state you're aiming for, and thus prep yourself according to its needs? What methods do you have at your disposal which will allow you to increase the chances of getting pregnant faster, or in keeping with your family plan?

These are the questions that this book has set out to answer.

So, are you ready to embark upon this journey to parenthood? To keep every tip and trick at your fingertips which could improve your chances of a quick conception, soon after you begin trying?

If so, let's get started!

Chapter 1: The Pre-Conception Preparations

While everyone who reaches the stage where they realize they're ready to have a child - wants to start right away, it's recommended by fertility experts that you give yourself a month or two to prepare your body accordingly so as to give yourselves the best chance of conception.

This period of pre-conception is important to wean yourselves off of any unhealthy habits, and to get your biological system as much on track as possible.

1] <u>Booze, Smokes & Drugs</u> - The first thing you should start with is to stop smoking, drinking, or taking drugs right away. While everyone and their mother knows this piece of advice, people only start following it **after** they've found out they're pregnant, and not before. However, if you're attempting to speed up your chances of conception, you should know that all of the above can get in the way of getting pregnant to begin with. Also, your fertilized egg is already attached to your uterus by the time you realize you're pregnant, and the soon-to-be-embryo is getting exposed to everything you're putting in your body. This will already have increased the chances of birth defects to a certain extent.

The drugs that I mention also include caffeine, just to be clear. Studies have already established a link between high caffeine consumption and decreased fertility, and – in some rare cases – chances of miscarriage. While there are conflicting reports on what may be considered a safe amount of caffeine to consume during pregnancy, it may be better to limit yourself to a maximum of 200mg of caffeine per day, though the best solution overall would be to kick the habit for now.

2] <u>Folic Acid</u> – Fertility experts state that regular consumption of Folic acid from a month before conception is crucial to reducing the risk of neutral-tube birth defects such as spina bifida by 50 to 70%, as researched by the CDC, and other birth defects to a lesser degree as well. The recommended minimum dosage is said to be 400 mcg per day, but dosages exceeding that wouldn't harm you either. In fact, in cases where the mother suffers from chronic diseases, and is on medication for them, the doses of Folic acid recommended by their doctors are much higher to prevent their medications causing birth defects.

If you're taking multivitamins with Folic acid to meet this requirement, make sure that your multivitamin doesn't contain more than the 770mcg daily recommended dose of vitamin A, unless most of it is present as beta-carotene, since a certain kind of vitamin A is known to be linked with higher chances of birth defects.

3] <u>Weight Issues</u> – Studies have shown that women may have an easier time conceiving if they're at a healthy weight. For some women, being at a higher or lower body mass index than the healthy range (below 20 or above 24) makes conception significantly more difficult.

Thus, it's for the best if – during this pre-conception period – you calculate your BMI and boost or reduce your weight as

10

necessary. It would make things significantly easier for you later on.

4] <u>Healthy Foods Galore</u> – While you may not be pregnant already, most of the eating habits that we have picked up in this modern age of ours affect fertility, conception and pregnancy greatly. It is thus recommended by fertility experts that you should start making smarter choices in your food and nutrition habits early, so that your body is stocked up on all the nutrients it requires to supply the fetus with, once you do conceive.

If nothing else, try eating at least 2 ½ cups of vegetables, as well as 2 cups of fruits, every day. Eschew refined flours, and switch over to whole grains. Make foods that are high in Calcium, as well as a variety of protein sources like beans, soy products, poultry and meats, a regular part of your diet. Even though the link here is tenuous, give preference to whole milk over skimmed milk, since whole milk is reputed to increase fertility over skimmed milk.

It is important that you pay special attention to the fish that you eat. While fish is an excellent source of omega-3 fatty acids – very important for a baby's eye and brain development – as well as vitamin D, protein and other essential nutrients, fish that may contain mercury may adversely affect the health of your fetus.

There are several lists of fish made available by experts online, which enumerate those which you should avoid during conception and pregnancy, including swordfish, king mackerel, and no more than 6 ounces of white canned tuna per week. The FDA recommends that pregnant women should eat up to 12 ounces a week of fish which have been listed as pregnancy-safe, like herring, salmon, sardines, etc. Always know the provenance of the fish you buy, it's safer to avoid fish caught in local water-bodies until you know the water is free of contaminants.

Stay away from unpasteurized cheeses, cold deli meats, and raw or undercooked fish and poultry. Any of these foods, and more besides, can carry dangerous bacteria which may lead to infections – which you need to avoid in the pre-conception period and thereafter. They could harm your baby-to-be.

5] <u>Reduce and Remove Risks In Your Environment</u> – While it may not be possible to entirely make your environment risk-free, this is the best time to assess what things around you pose a risk to the development and birth of your child. If you feel like your job is hazardous to a child, that you are exposed to radiation or harmful chemicals on a daily basis, you may have to make some changes soon in that regard.

While some people overlook this part, please do not forget that even household items like cleaning liquids, pesticides, insecticides, etc. are harmful for the development of an unborn child, and you may either need to switch to safer products, or figure out ways to minimize your exposure to them.

6] Establish An Exercise Routine – The most effective way of getting your body to the best possible pre-conception state is by deciding on and **enforcing** an exercise routine right away! The healthier you are before you get pregnant, the less the complications you may be likely to face during or after. You could start by walking for half an hour every day, or by adding more exercise to your already-established work routine, like taking the stairs instead of the elevator.

Not only will this help you get ready for having a baby inside you, it will also act as a great stress buster. The endorphins you release while working up that sweat are top-of-the-line mood up-lifters, and the best part is that they're self-supplied!

7] All Hail the Super Sperm! – It would be wrong to assume that the mother-to-be is the only one who has to make pre-conception preps in order to be at her best before you get down to conceiving. Sperms have to be healthy, active and strong so that they can last longer and reach your fallopian tubes to fertilize the egg.

It is important for the father-to-be to start avoiding hot tubs, hot baths and saunas, since the excessive heat kills sperm.

It's just as important for the father-to-be to stop smoking or consuming recreational drugs as well, as these are known to cause poor sperm function.

The father-to-be also has to get his store of nutrients ready in order to make strong, healthy sperm. For this reason, consumption of supplements like zinc, calcium, vitamin C and Folic acid becomes of paramount importance in this pre-conception time and beyond.

8] <u>On To Medical Matters / Pre-Conception Visit</u> – While you may pursue a lot of preparations yourselves, all of it may lead nowhere without a pre-conception visit to your doctor or Ob-Gyn.

Once you and your partner are mentally ready to conceive, schedule the visit with your respective doctor as early as possible. Before you go, make sure that you're updated on any congenital diseases or other maladies that your genes may place your child at a higher risk of.

Your doctor should then review both of your personal and family medical histories, your present states of health, and any medication that the mother-to-be may be on, which may hamper conception or pregnancy. He will then be able to make modifications as necessary. In some cases you will still have to wait a while before you try conceiving –some drugs are stored in your body fat and take longer to expel from your body.

If you've been on methods of birth control other than physical barriers, i.e. birth control pills, etc. you may need to ask the doctor about how long you need to wait after you've stopped taking them for your eggs to start dropping normally again. While, in most cases, doctors recommend waiting till your period cycles have regularized again after you've stopped the pills – usually a month or two after you've ceased all internal forms of birth control – in the case of some pills it could take a year before the eggs start dropping normally – even if your periods have already been regular for a while.

Your doctor will also have to check your diet, weight, and physical fitness issues; recommend which supplements and multivitamins you put yourself on; check if you're up-to-date on immunizations; test your immunity to childhood diseases such as chicken-pox; test couples who may want to undergo genetic testing for specific conditions their child may be at risk of from either of the families; conduct fertility tests if needed (though they usually aren't at this point, unless there is something specific in the background medical histories), etc.

You could also take your doctor through your daily routines, and materials you regularly come in contact with, to get their advice on hazards, chemical or otherwise, and how to reduce them. Also consider visiting your dentist for a check-up in this period. The hormonal shifts that occur during pregnancy sometimes exacerbate gum diseases that were slowly developing, kicking them into high-gear. Taking care of this matter during your pre-conception should effectively reduce the risks of any such occurrence later on.

Once you believe you're well prepared with regards to your pre-conception health and needs, you can move on to the next part.

Chapter 2: It's Ovulation Time!

After you've cleared everything with your doctor, you've finished your pre-conception preparations, and you're certain that your eggs are now dropping normally – the next step to conception is figuring out your ovulation period.

The duration of a woman's menstrual cycle is actually quite varied, ranging from 21 days to as much as 35 days, with 28 days the average. Ovulation is the part of the cycle where the egg is released from the ovaries, out of the 15 to 20 eggs maturing in them. The ripest egg, or eggs in some cases, is the one that's ultimately released into the fallopian tube. This part of the cycle is usually a 4 to 6 day period, and only signals a singular release of egg(s), which is why it's important to know when you're ovulating. This is the only period of time where sex can lead to fertilization, and then in turn to conception.

If the egg is fertilized thereafter, it descends and attaches itself to the wall of the uterus, and starts its development to an embryo. If it is not fertilized within 24 hours, then the egg disintegrates and dissolves before reaching the uterus, eventually triggering the shedding of the uterine wall during a woman's period or menses later in the menstrual cycle. The whole process then repeats itself.

There are a few ways that I'll discuss here, ranging from the easiest to the most accurate, as to how you can figure out when you're ovulating. Some of these depend on your periods occurring with some regularity – in terms of their occurrences as well the length of the cycle. However, if your periods are really irregular, i.e. occurring twice in a three-month period, etc. it may be best for you to take the help of your doctor.

1] <u>Counting the Days</u> – While an old-fashioned method, and the easiest of the following, counting the days depend on the mother-to-be having her periods with some regularity.

The first step is to figure out on what days of the months your last two or three periods occured. Use that to determine when you think your next period will start. (Just to be clear: Day 1 is the first day of this period, while the last day is when the menses of this period will end and before the day 1 of the next period will start)

Once you have an idea of the date when your next period will start, count back 12 days, and then another four. Your ovulation will most likely occur during this 4 to 5-day range. If you have your periods with regularity, and are one of those whose period length falls across the 28-day average, there may be a good chance that you'll ovulate on day 14 of your cycle.

2] <u>Listen to Your Body</u> – Between this method and the previous one, this particular technique gives you a more accurate reading of when you might be ovulating. However, to understand your body and its signals, you'll need a month or two of preparing and observing before you can use it with enough certainty to be able to use it to determine when you're ovulating.

What you need to do is to track the changes in your Basal Body Temperature – the lowest body temperature in a 24-hour period – and your vaginal discharge.

While the change may be too small for you to notice, a few days after you ovulate, your BBT rises. However, this rise is maybe a difference of 0.5 – 1.0 degree Fahrenheit, and that's why you need to observe yourself for a month or two before you can use it to determine your ovulation period.

The second difference you can track is your vaginal discharge. During the normal course of the month, most women usually have very little cervical mucus discharging from their vagina. However, as they approach ovulation, the cervical mucus changes in terms of texture and quantity – becoming more slippery, clear and stretchy.

While one of these two factors alone may make for a very shaky prediction, the two of them tracked together over the course of a month or two – enough for you to understand the signals your own body is giving you – may help you to make significantly more accurate predictions regarding your ovulation from the third cycle.

3] **Hormone Testing** – Out of all the ways that we have discussed, the most accurate one of them by far is using an Ovulation Predictor Kit.

This is a pee-on-a-stick test kit which checks your hormone

levels, and gives you a positive result on the day **before** you ovulate. This essentially works by testing your level of Luteinizing Hormone, and if it goes up. When the LH goes up, you get a positive test, and it means one of your ovaries will soon release an egg.

While these may be a bit on the expensive side, they're quite accurate and can be bought over-the-counter without any need for a prescription.

Once you and your partner have figured out a rough or accurate window of ovulation in your cycle, it's time to hit the sheets!

Chapter 3: Getting Busy. And Liking It.

Now that you have your ovulation window clear in your head, and the science experiment is over, it's time to have some fun with the practicals.

And before you think I'm being overly flippant about the 'having fun' part, studies have already shown that if the couple trying to conceive is stressed about it, the process isn't as effective. The hypothalamus, which regulates the hormones of ovulation, doesn't function as well under stress, which could drastically affect when and *if* you'll ovulate in that cycle. So, having fun with your sex life while trying to conceive, rather than becoming Robo-BabyMakers V1.0, is proven to boost your chances of pregnancy greatly.

With your ovulation window in mind, the best way to increase the chances of success is to start having sex from three days before the start of the ovulation period, till the day after you suspect it's done.

While the egg can only survive in your fallopian tube for about a day, sperms can last and wait for the egg for three to six days in your body. Also, it's important to make sure that if you and your partner haven't had sex in a while, he should ejaculate at least once in the days before your period of highest fertility. Otherwise, the sperm in his built-up semen could be dead, which wouldn't fertilize the egg either way.

If you are unsure of when your ovulation period falls exactly, the easiest way to circumvent it is to have sex at least every alternate day during the suspected time. This way, when your egg does drop, there will always be a supply of healthy sperm waiting in your tubes to fertilize it.

Just to bust a myth here, no particular sexual position is more effective than any other at increasing the chances of conception. However, studies have proven that simply lying on your back for 15-20 minutes after you have been inseminated by your partner could increase your chances of conception by as much as 50%.

Chapter 4: How Long to Wait Before Seeking Help

Without raining on anyone's parade, most couples nowadays start freaking out if they haven't conceived within the first two months of trying. However, you need to relax and give yourselves some time.

For about 6 out of 10 couples who are trying to get pregnant naturally, conception usually occurs within the first three months. However, if you don't fit in that number, you shouldn't start panicking or stressing, especially since that will hamper rather than help the process anyway. Almost half of the others in that number of couples trying to conceive are in the same boat as you. It's normal and natural for some to take longer than others in this matter.

If you're under the age of 35, with no known fertility issues in all the visits that you and your partner have shared with the doctor in the pre-conception period, at least give yourselves 8 months to a year before you think about seeking professional help in the matter.

Conception is one of the most beautiful, intricate and complex natural processes in the known world. The smallest stress that you may be feeling may be throwing you off. You and your partner need to relax, believe in each other, remember that no matter what you'd go through it together, and keep having fun in the bedroom while continuing your normal lives – how hard does that really sound?

If you're between the ages of 35 to 40, you should keep in mind that fertility decreases after a point with age, and should consider seeking help after 6 months of trying without results.

As for those of you who are above the age of 40, it might be best to involve fertility testing in your pre-conception period so that your doctors can advise you on any hormone or fertility therapy that may be required in case you have issues.

Beyond these pointers, if you've followed the tips I laid out in the pre-conception preparations, and are still within the time periods I spelt out above, relax and enjoy your lives and your partners till the said time period passes.

I understand that the stress is normal, and it may sometimes be frustrating, but you need to believe in yourselves just a little longer. If none of the tests that you took had any cause for alarm, then all that it may take is a little time and patience.

Switch to yoga, meditation, more adventurous sex if that suits your needs, or any other activities which may further help you manage that stress, as I've already explained the link between stress and fertility before.

If, even after all that, you have trouble conceiving, then seek professional help without hesitation.

Chapter 5: Natural Herbs as Fertility Boosters

While there are plenty of powders, strange-smelling liquids and other such products that are touted as miracle fertility boosters, the truth is that few of them really are. While you may not have the time, patience, energy or conviction to sit and research them all, I can at least provide you with a few known, nourishing natural supplements which may help you, to a greater or lesser degree, improve your health and, through it, boost your fertility.

1] Royal Jelly: A creamy substance produced by bees to nourish their queen in her task of laying eggs for the hive, Royal Jelly is a rich source of amino acids, sugars, vitamins, lipids, fatty acids and proteins. It also contains much-needed iron and calcium in abundance. The consumption of Royal Jelly has been shown to help in balancing bodily hormonal functions.

2] Maca: This is a Peruvian root which has been shown to support hormonal balance. It contains 60 different plant-derived nutrients and 31 different minerals. It acts as a nourishing food for the endocrine system, which is paramount in hormonal balance and regulation.

3] Spirulina: A cyanobacteria, more commonly known as blue - green algae, spirulina is considered to be the highest-quality plant protein source. This bacterium also provides a treasure-trove of vitamins and minerals.

4] Dandelion Leaf: A nourishing natural supplement, the dandelion leaf is used to right nutritional imbalances and helps in supporting the liver, which further improves hormonal balance.

5] Lemon Balm Leaf: This leaf is excellent nourishment for the nervous system. It promotes healthier stress responses and lessens depression and anxiety, which is vital for those aiming to conceive. This is not to be used by people with hypothyroidism though.

6] Red Raspberry Leaf: This leaf is highly nutritious, and is high in vitamins and minerals. Most importantly, it serves as a uterine tonic which helps in preparing the uterus for pregnancy and labor.

7] Seaweed (Agar, Arame, Wakame, etc.): Safely cultivated and packaged seaweed is extremely high in vitamins and minerals, including iodine, which is paramount for thyroid function. Some varieties of Seaweed also help to improve estrogen metabolism.

8] Wild Yam Root (Dioscorea villosa): This root is known to promote healthier menstrual cycles, and to reduce ovarian pain.

9] Vitex or Chaste Tree Berry (Vitex agnus-castus): This berry is known to improve the timing of menstrual cycles, promote ovulation, and help in regulating hormonal balance.

While there are many more of such natural boosters present in nature, do not buy or use one simply at face value. If you come across more such natural products, be sure to read up all you can about them and their ingredients. Since, like any other good thing, too much may do more harm than good, ensure that you don't exceed suggested dosages or bypass the recommended methods of use. In case of any confusion or doubt, be sure to consult your doctor before you start using any potent natural product, so as to avoid possible interactions or harmful effects.

While using natural products is a good way of boosting your health and fertility yourselves, do not forget that almost every drug out there was derived from, synthesized through, or artificially created based on a drug found in such natural plants all around us. If used without proper knowledge, they **do** wreak just as much harm as good. But no, this doesn't necessarily apply to the herbal green tea you're sipping on right now while reading this, though that too depends on its ingredients.

Conclusion

Although conception is one of the most fun natural processes out there, predating a big change like parenthood, several couples get impatient soon after they begin to attempt. They then get stressed, then depressed, then they either blame themselves or each other, when all they had to do was have fun, and be a little more patient.

While there are undeniably those who do end up needing professional help, do not assume anything before you know for sure. Under no circumstances should this beautiful period in your life be a source of strain, though strain, stress and frustration is only normal if we give in and give up.

Keep your partner close throughout your period of conception. Remember that you love and cherish each other, and that's why you've decided to expand your family to begin with. In most cases, everything will go off without a hitch, given an appropriate amount of time. And even if it doesn't, while it may be a little saddening, there are a hundred different ways from here on out that we haven't even discussed, and that you haven't attempted yet. One way or another, as long as you stay happily beside each other, and keep the core of your new family strong, one day you'll have the growing, exuberant, happy family you've always wanted.

Keep your thoughts on happier matters. Congratulations on reaching this joyous phase in what will surely be a long and prosperous life.

In the end – Always keep trying. After all, how can even more sex ever be a bad thing? And how can something really worth having in your life just drop into your lap without trying?

Finally, I'd like to thank you for purchasing this book! If you enjoyed it or found it helpful, I'd greatly appreciate it if you'd take a moment to leave a review on Amazon. Thanks, and good luck!

Manufactured by Amazon.ca
Bolton, ON

26016039R00022